Health
Organizer

A Personal Health-Care Record

Published by

ARTHRITIS FOUNDATION®

Take Control. We Can Help.™

Published by
Arthritis Foundation
1330 West Peachtree Street NW
Suite 100
Atlanta, Georgia 30309

Printed in Canada

Foreword

Communicating well with your doctors is essential to managing your health. One of the best ways you can do this is by keeping track of your health and informing your doctor of any changes you notice. By keeping your doctor informed of your symptoms and progress, you can play an active role in your health care. Working together, you and your doctor can find the most effective ways to manage your health.

In this book, we've provided you with a clear system for organizing all of the information about your health. Each section is designed to help you track specific information, such as diagnoses, medications, surgeries and daily progress. Together, these sections make this book a central place for all of your health-related information. This tool will also allow you to chart the changes in your health over time, noting symptoms that worsen as well as therapies or exercises that make your feel better. Then, when you visit your doctor you'll have a detailed record that will help your doctor to evaluate your progress and work with you to develop an appropriate management plan. Using this organizer will help you better understand your condition and will give you a sense of increased control over your health.

So pick up a pen and begin using your Arthritis Foundation Health Organizer now. We hope you find it gives you insight into your condition and that it serves as a springboard for discussions and partnership with your doctor in managing your health.

Patience White, MD
Chief Public Health Officer
Arthritis Foundation

Introduction

Congratulations on choosing this health organizer. It means that you have made a decision to take control of your arthritis and your health.

If you have recently received an arthritis diagnosis, you may feel overwhelmed by all of information you are receiving — or you may wonder where you can find more information. If you've had arthritis awhile, you know that managing your disease can be lifelong job, which at times can also be overwhelming.

Managing your arthritis — and your health — involves understanding your disease, knowing your treatment options, assembling a health-care team and knowing how to communicate with your team members so that your needs are met. It also means following through with treatment recommendations and making healthy lifestyle choices, such as exercising, eating well, maintaining a healthy weight, managing stress and getting enough sleep. That's a lot to remember and keep up with. This book can help.

How to Use This Book

This organizer is divided into the following eight sections that can help you take a greater role in managing your arthritis by providing important, basic information about some of the most common forms of arthritis and related conditions and an easy to way record and organize your health information.

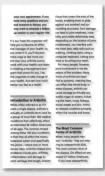

1 Introduction to Arthritis

The first step for anyone in managing a medical problem is to learn as much as possible about their disease. In this introductory section, we'll help you get started with a brief overview of some of the most common forms of arthritis and related conditions and some common questions and concerns about them. We'll also offer some tips on how to use this book — your own personal health

organizer — to better manage your arthritis and your health.

2 Record Keeper

This section is designed as a place to record your general health information and medical history. You'll find spaces designated for names, phone numbers, addresses of your health-care team members and the health facilities you use; your insurance company and policy information; and

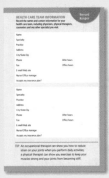

How to Use This Book

details about your personal medical history. The Record Keeper section will be a ready reference for you, a place where you can consolidate information about your health background.

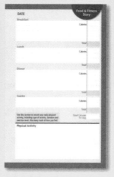

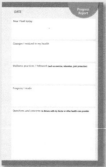

3 Progress Report

In this section, you'll keep periodic updates on your health. You can track your symptoms, medication side effects, questions, and even emotional events, such as stress, that affect your health. Looking over these notes before doctor's appointments can help you remember concerns you want to discuss with your doctor. And the details about how you've been feeling will help your doctor determine the proper treatment for you. Use the back of the page to take notes at your appointment.

4 Food & Fitness Diary

In this section, you can track your meals and daily physical activity. Use it to count calories and to assess your exertion level and how you feel when you exercise.

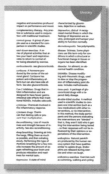

5 Glossary

We've include definitions of almost 200 terms commonly used in the diagnosis and treatment of arthritis. Knowing these words will help you feel more at ease discussing your condition.

How to Use This Book

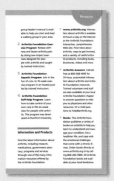

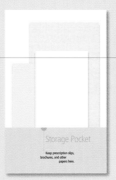

6 Resources

Here you'll find an overview of useful services and products offered by the Arthritis Foundation.

8 Storage Pocket

The Storage Pocket gives you a place to keep all those stray pieces of paper you may acquire, such as prescription slips, appointment reminders, business cards and brochures. You can even file health-related newspaper or magazine articles to discuss with your physician during your appointment.

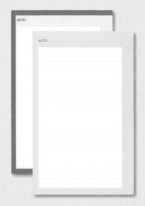

7 Notes

Use these blank pages throughout the book to write down additional information, resources or questions, or to take notes at your office visits.

Getting Started

Keeping this kind of health organizer will be somewhat different from writing your thoughts and feelings in the typical journals you may be familiar with. As a new experience, it may take some time to feel comfortable. But if you stick with it, you'll have a valuable tool for managing your health.

Because a series of blank pages can be daunting at first, try starting your journal by filling in the health information you already know, such as your physician's name and contact information, your insurance company and your medical history. Then start your Progress Report by writing what you think is important about your health and how you feel. The pages include a few general questions to guide you in thinking about your health. Here are some ways you can begin your organizer and make it as useful as possible:

- Don't worry about misspellings or the quality of your writing. Try using short phrases and lists for a simple, quick way to write your thoughts.

- Date your entries so you can easily see the patterns and progress in your health.

- Note specifics about your health, such as symptom fluctuations, unusual symptoms, medication side effects, diet, activities, self-care practices and stress or positive changes in your condition.

- Use descriptive words in your entries (for example, write something like "sharp" or "hot" when describing pain) to help you remember the feeling and explain it to your doctor later. Carefully describing how you feel will help you notice the differences in your symptoms.

- Don't feel obligated to write in the journal every day. Focusing too much on the details of the illness can keep you from concentrating on wellness.

- Ask for advice on what information your doctor needs from you. Keep track of that information in the Record Keeper section.

- Write down questions you have for your doctor—as you think of them.

- Look over your notes to determine how much time you'll need with your doctor during

your next appointment. If you have many questions and several concerns to discuss, you may want to schedule a follow-up session to your regular visit.

It is our hope this organizer will help you to become an effective manager of your health. As you write in it, you'll discover more ways to feel more control over your arthritis and to work with your health-care team in creating a management program that works for you. Use this organizer to take charge of your health. And see how much better you feel as a result!

Introduction to Arthritis

While often referred to as if it were a single disease, arthritis is actually an umbrella term used for a group of more than 100 medical conditions that collectively affect an estimated 46 million Americans of all ages. The common thread among these 100-plus conditions is that they all affect the musculoskeletal system and specifically the joints—where two or more bones meet. Arthritis-related joint problems include pain, stiffness, inflammation and damage to joint cartilage (the tough, smooth

tissue that covers the ends of the bones, enabling them to glide against one another) and surrounding structures. Such damage can lead to joint weakness, instability and visible deformities that, depending on the location of joint involvement, can interfere with the most basic daily tasks such as walking, climbing stairs, using a computer keyboard, cutting your food or brushing your teeth.

For many people, however, joint involvement is not the extent of the problem. Many forms of arthritis are classified as systemic, meaning they can affect the whole body. In these diseases, arthritis can cause damage to virtually any bodily organ or system, including the heart, lungs, kidneys, blood vessels and skin. Arthritis-related conditions primarily affect the muscles and bones.

The Most Common Forms of Arthritis

Osteoarthritis
When many people mention "arthritis," they are referring to Osteoarthritis (OA). The most common form of the disease, OA affects an estimated

27 million Americans.

If you have osteoarthritis, you probably experience morning stiffness and mild to moderate pain that may come on slowly throughout the day or may come and go periodically. On the other hand, you may have pain and stiffness that steadily worsen, making it difficult to go about your daily life.

The pain of OA is usually in or around the affected joint, which most commonly are those of the knees, hips, fingers neck and lower back. If osteoarthritic joint changes cause pressure on the nerves and muscles surrounding the joint, the pain may be felt elsewhere, a problem known as referred pain.

Deformities due to overgrowth of bone at the margins of the joint are common in osteoarthritis, particularly the fingers. Knobby bone growths called Heberden's nodes (in the joint nearest the nail) or Bouchard's nodes (in the joint in the middle of the finger) may appear on one finger or several fingers. They may cause chronic or intermittent pain and interfere with the ability to enjoy such leisure activities as needlework, playing the piano or golfing.

Other common forms of arthritis are:

Rheumatoid Arthritis

The second most common form of arthritis, rheumatoid arthritis affects an estimated 1.3 million Americans. Although it can occur in people of any age, most cases are diagnosed in people between 30 and 50.

The pain of RA is caused by inflammation of the synovium, the thin membrane that lines the joint. Inflammation can be so severe that it damages cartilage, bone and connective tissue. Joint involvement in RA is usually symmetrical. That is, if one elbow or knee is inflamed and painful, the other elbow or knee likely will be. The joints RA is most likely to affect are those of the fingers, hands, wrists, elbows, shoulders, knees, ankles and feet. In rare cases, RA can also affect the skin, muscles, and internal organs such as the heart and lungs.

Fibromyalgia

The most common arthritis-related condition, fibromyalgia does not affect the joints. Instead, fibromyalgia is characterized by widespread pain and fatigue and the presence of tender points, or specific areas of the body that are particularly painful upon the application of the slightest pressure. Other problems associated with fibromyalgia include headaches; difficulty concentrating; irritable bowel syndrome and pain or dysfunction with the temporomandibular joints (TMJ), which attach the lower jaw to the skull on each side of the face.

Ankylosing Spondylitis

Ankylosing Spondylitis (AS) is one of a group of diseases collectively referred to as the spondylarthropathies, a term that means arthritis that affects the spine. Typically these diseases attack the sacroiliac joints that attach the spine to the pelvis and the stack of bones called the vertebrae, which form the spinal column. Other common features of these diseases include arthritis in other joints (commonly, the shoulder, hips, knees and ankles) and involvement of other tissues including those of the skin, eyes, bowel and genitourinary tract.

Gout

Gout occurs when a bodily waste product called uric acid builds up in the body and crystallizes in the joints, causing severe pain and inflammation. Gout usually strikes a single joint suddenly. Inflammation and swelling of the affected joint may be so severe that the skin over the joint is pulled taut and appears shiny and red or purplish.

Typically, inflammation subsides on its own within a week or so. However, unless the high level of uric acid is treated, attacks will return with increasing frequency and affect more joints, including the feet, knees and elbows. If allowed to progress, gout can lead to joint damage.

Lupus

Systemic lupus erythematosus (SLE), often referred to simply as lupus, is an inflammatory disease that affects an estimated 250,000 Americans. It affects six times as many women as men and four times as many African Americans as Caucasians. It is most likely to begin during a woman's childbearing years.

Like other forms of arthritis, lupus causes inflammation of the joints, typically those of the hands, wrists, elbows, knees and feet. But it can also affect the skin, blood, lungs, kidneys and cardiovascular and nervous systems. Treatment is essential not only to ease symptoms but to prevent organ damage.

Other arthritis-related conditions include:

- **osteoporosis, a condition in which the body loses so much bone mass that bones are susceptible to disabling fractures after the slightest trauma**

- **polymyositis, a disease of generalized weakness that results from inflammation of the muscles**

- **scleroderma, a disease that results from an overgrowth of collagen within the skin. In some forms of the disease, the effects of this abnormal overgrowth are limited to the skin and underlying tissues. In others, connective tissue build-up can affect the function of the joints, blood vessels and internal organs.**

- **polymyalgia rheumatica, a disease in which inflammation in the joints of the neck, shoulder and hip areas causes stiffness and aching in those areas. It mainly affects older people.**

What Causes Arthritis?

There are probably many causes of arthritis, which differ by the type of arthritis.

Osteoarthritis, for example, is caused by the breakdown of joint cartilage. This can occur as the result of genetic defects in cartilage, congenital abnormalities in joint alignment, joint injuries or overuse and obesity.

Weight has also shown to be a factor in gout, which occurs when excess uric acid in the bloodstream seeps out into the tissues and forms crystals.

For many inflammatory forms of arthritis, such as rheumatoid arthritis and lupus, the disease is the result of an aberrant immune response. In these diseases, the immune system, which is designed to protect the body against invaders, mistakenly attacks the body's healthy tissues. Although no one knows exactly what causes the immune system to go awry, scientists suspect a combination of genetic and environmental factors.

Already, a number of genes for various diseases—including rheumatoid arthritis and lupus—have been identified. Some link these diseases to other autoimmune diseases.

Many researchers are working

to find the cause of the different forms of arthritis in the hope that a better understanding of the causes will lead to ways to prevent the diseases or improve their treatment.

Diagnosing Arthritis

If you suspect you have arthritis, but have not seen a doctor about it, it's important that you do so as soon as possible. If you have an inflammatory form of the disease such as rheumatoid arthritis, the earlier you receive a diagnosis and begin treatment, the better your chances are of controlling the disease and preventing joint damage and disability. For all diseases, getting a diagnosis and the right treatment can help relieve symptoms and help you feel better.

In general, you should consult a doctor if you experience arthritis symptoms that come on suddenly, such as a joint rapidly becoming hot, swollen or difficult to move, or if you have any of the following symptoms for longer than two weeks:

- **Pain in a joint that doesn't go away or keeps returning**
- **Joint stiffness**
- **Swelling in a joint, especially with warmth and redness**
- **Joint or muscle pain accompanied by fatigue, malaise or fever**

If you have begun the diagnostic process, but don't have an answer yet, stick with it—and be patient. Sometimes determining the form of arthritis you have can be long process. (Fortunately, your doctor can in many cases begin effective treatment before the precise disease is identified.) Unlike diabetes or kidney disease, arthritis cannot be diagnosed with a simple blood test. Instead, the diagnosis is based largely on what the doctor hears from you (the medical history) and observes in you (the physical exam).

During the medical history, your doctor will ask questions about specific joints as well as how you feel in general. Because findings from the medical history play a major role in the diagnosis, it's important to give your doctor clear and accurate and answers to any questions she asks. You should also be prepared to tell the doctor the following:

- **When the pain started**
- **What the pain feels like**
- **How long the pain lasts**
- **What time of day the pain is worst**

- Other symptoms you've noticed
- Other medical conditions you have
- Childhood illnesses you've had
- Adult illnesses you've had
- Surgeries you've had
- Injuries you've had
- Lifestyle habits (good and bad)
- Medical conditions your family members have had

Along with the medical history, a thorough physical exam will supply most of the information needed to make the diagnosis. Things your doctor will look for in the exam include:

- Joint swelling, warmth and redness
- Joint tenderness
- Loss of motion in your joints
- Joints that are out of alignment
- Signs of disease involvement in other organs, such as the heart, lungs or kidneys

After the medical history and physical examination, your doctor may order lab tests and imaging procedures to help confirm your diagnosis. These tests include:

- **Erythrocyte sedimentation rate (sed rate)**, a blood test that measures the rate at which red blood cells sink and form sediment in the bottom of a test tube. An elevated rate indicates inflammation.

- **C-reactive protein**, a measure of inflammation that indicates disease activity

- **Uric acid**, a bodily waste product. Abnormally high levels may indicate gout.

- **Rheumatoid factor**, an antibody found in the blood of about 70 to 80 percent of people with RA

- **Antinuclear antibodies (ANA)**, antibodies that combine with the nuclei of cells and appear in about 95 percent of people with lupus and smaller percentages of people with RA and some other arthritis-related conditions.

- **Anti-CCP antibody**, an antibody that binds to the amino acid citrulline, which is present in most people with rheumatoid arthritis. When the antibody is found in the blood, there a 90 percent or greater likelihood that a person has RA.

- **X-rays**, which can show swelling of soft tissues, irregularities in joint cartilage, bony changes in the spine and loss of bone density around affected joints

- **Magnetic resonance imaging (MRI),** which can show synovitis, inflammation of the joint lining, before damage shows up on X-ray, as well as inflammation in other organs

- **Ultrasonography,** the use of sound waves to produce pictures of structures within the body

- **Biopsies,** the examination of pieces of bodily tissue that are removed surgically. Depending on the piece of tissue removed, your doctor may use a biopsy to diagnose diseases of the joint, muscle skin or blood vessels.

- **Arthroscopy,** a surgical procedure in which a lighted scope is inserted into the joint through a small incision. The scope is attached to a close-circuit television, which, allowing the doctor to see and possible diagnose problems in the joint.

Later, some of these same tests may be used to monitor the progress of your disease and/ or its response to treatment.

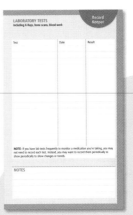

How You Can Use This Organizer:

Use the Laboratory Test pages in the Record Keeper section of this book to keep track of these tests and their results. Use the Progress Report pages to jot down any questions you have concerning test results or further tests you need.

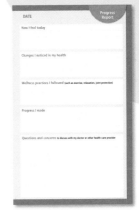

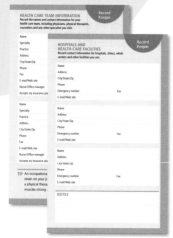

Who Treats Arthritis?

Treating arthritis may require a team of health-care professionals rather than one doctor. Professionals such as physical therapists, occupational therapists, pharmacists and nurses can all play an important role in the management of your disease.

In most cases your primary doctor for arthritis should be a rheumatologist. A rheumatologist is an internist (a doctor who specializes in internal medicine and treating adult diseases) who has additional training to diagnose and treat arthritis or related diseases that affect the joints, muscles, bones, skin and other tissues. Some rheumatologists may also have special training in pediatrics, orthopaedics, physical medicine, sports medicine or other medical fields.

While a rheumatologist is the best doctor to manage your arthritis, you will still need a primary care physician to manage other aspects of your health care. Unfortunately, having arthritis doesn't make you immune to other health problems. In fact, certain forms of arthritis share risk factors with other diseases. In some forms of arthritis, other health problems can occur as a result of the disease or its treatment. (See "Arthritis and the Risk of Other Diseases")

Communicating with Your Doctor

Good communication with your doctor is essential to getting the best care for your RA. One of the best ways to improve your communication with your doctor is to prepare for your appointments ahead of time. Consider these tips when getting ready for your visit:

- **Look over notes you've made in your Health Organizer since your last appointment. Take note of any patterns or changes in your health that you need to discuss.**

- **Make note of the progress you've made in managing your arthritis and think through your concerns so you can update your doctor.**

- **Choose three or four of your most important concerns to discuss first during the appointment.**

- **Make a note of prescriptions you need refilled.**

- **Consider having medical or lab tests done in advance so you'll have the results to discuss at your appointment.**

- **Make a list of questions you would like to ask your doctor at your appointment. Questions could include: Which symptoms or changes I tolerate before calling you? What are my treatment options and how do they work? How long before a treatment takes effect? What are the potential side effects and what should I do about them? Are there other health professionals I should see, treatments I should try, exercises I should do and/or classes I should take?**

Before you leave your doctor's office, review the topics you've discussed to make sure you understand what was said. And be sure to find out what your doctor expects you to do before your next appointment, such as taking a new medication, following a certain exercise program or meeting a weight-loss goal.

How Arthritis Is Treated

Treatment for arthritis may consist of medications to ease symptoms, stop damaging inflammation and, in the case of rheumatoid arthritis, slow or stop the disease process.

There are many different drugs used in the treatment of arthritis. Some forms of arthritis and related conditions, such as fibromyalgia, gout and osteoporosis, are treated with medications that are rarely, if ever, used to treat other forms of the disease.

However, the drugs used for most forms of arthritis and related conditions fall into one of these categories:

Analgesics

Analgesics are medications that work purely to relieve pain. The most commonly used and readily available analgesic is acetaminophen (*Tylenol*). For many people, acetaminophen alone is sufficient to relieve OA pain. For more severe pain that doesn't respond to acetaminophen doctors may prescribe narcotic analgesics such as tramadol (*Ultram*), oxycodone (*OxyContin, Roxicodone*) or propoxyphene hydrochloride (*Darvon, PP-Cap*)

NSAIDs

Nonsteroidal anti-inflammatory drugs include more than a dozen different medications—some available over-the-counter, some available by prescription only—used to help ease arthritis pain and inflammation. NSAIDs include such drugs as ibuprofen (*Advil, Motrin*), ketoprofen (*Actron, Orudis KT*) and naproxen sodium (*Aleve*), among others. If you have had or are at risk of stomach ulcers, your doctor may prescribe celecoxib (*Celebrex*), a type of NSAID called a COX-2 inhibitor, which is designed to be safer for the stomach.

Corticosteroids

Corticosteroid medications, including prednisone, prednisolone and methyprednisolone, are potent and quick-acting anti-inflammatory medications. They may be used in RA to get potentially damaging inflammation under control, while waiting for NSAIDs and DMARDs (below) take effect. Because of the risk of side effects with these drugs, doctors prefer to use them for as short a time as possible and in doses as low as possible.

DMARDs

An acronym for disease-modifying antirheumatic drugs, DMARDs are drugs that work slowly to actually modify the course of the disease. In recent years, the most commonly used DMARD for rheumatoid arthritis is methotrexate. But there are about a dozen others that fall into this category. They include hydroxychloroquine (*Plaquenil*), sulfasalazine (*Azulfidine*, *Azulfidine EN-Tabs*), leflunomide (*Arava*) and azathioprine (*Imuran*). A person diagnosed with RA today is likely to be prescribed a DMARD fairly early in the course of their disease, as doctors have found that starting these drugs early on can help prevent irreparable joint damage that might occur if their use was delayed.

Biologic Agents

The newest category of medications used for rheumatoid arthritis is that of the biologic agents. There are currently six such agents approved for rheumatoid arthritis: abatacept (*Orencia*), adalimumab (*Humira*), anakinra (*Kineret*), etanercept (*Enbrel*), infliximab (*Remicade*) and rituximab (*Rituxan*). Each of the biologics blocks a specific step in the inflammation process. *Humira*, *Enbrel* and *Remicade* block a cytokine called tumor necrosis factor-alpha (TNF-α), and therefore often are called TNF-α inhibitors. *Kineret* blocks

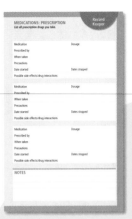

How You Can Use This Organizer:

Use the Medication sheets in the Record Keeper section to record the names and dosages of medications your doctor prescribes. Use the Progress Report to note any questions about medications you'd like to bring up at your next office visit.

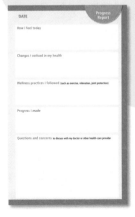

a cytokine called interleukin-1 (IL-1). Orencia blocks the activation of T cells. *Rituxan* blocks B cells. Because these agents target specific steps in the process, they don't wipe out the entire immune response as some other RA treatments do, and in many people a biologic agent can slow, modify or stop the disease—even when other treatments haven't helped much.

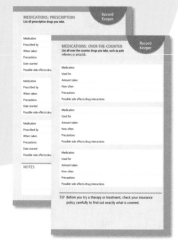

Medication Side Effects

All medications—even ones you buy without a prescription—have the potential for side effects. Arthritis medications are no exception. While some side effects are serious and necessitate discontinuing the medication, others may be alleviated by adjusting the dosage or timing of the drug or by taking another drug to offset the adverse effect (for example, taking an acid-blocking drug to help offset the stomach discomfort and ulcer risk caused by NSAIDs). Sometimes side effects go away after a while, or you may find them worth enduring in return for the benefits you receive from a drug. If you suspect you are experiencing a drug side effect, contact your doctor before stopping the medication.

It's also possible for the medications you take for arthritis to interact negatively with medications prescribed for other medical conditions or even with some foods or beverages, particularly alcoholic ones. In some cases, these interactions can be minimized or eliminated by spacing out two medications. In others, switching medications—or avoiding medications with potential for interaction to begin with—may be necessary.

It is impossible to list all of the side effects for arthritis medication because different drugs cause different side effects and different people react differently to medications. But the following are some of the more common ones:

- **Analgesics**—**Constipation, dizziness, nausea, potential for psychological and physical dependence (narcotic analgesics only). Other side effects vary by drug.**

- **Nonsteroidal anti-inflammatory drugs (NSAIDs)**—**Edema (swelling of the feet), heartburn, stomach upset and stomach ulcers and possibly increased risk of blood clots,** heart attack and stroke.

- **Corticocosteroids**—**Cataracts, elevated blood fats and blood sugar levels, increased appetite and bone loss.**

- **Disease-modifying antirheumatic drugs (DMARDs)**—**Stomach upset and increased susceptibility to infection. Other side effects vary by drug.**

- **Biologic agents**—**Injection or infusion site reactions, including redness and swelling, and increased risk of serious infections. Other side effects vary by drug.**

Natural Supplements for Arthritis

People who are frustrated with conventional arthritis medications for may be attracted to herbs, supplements and other natural remedies.

While natural treatments are appealing, it's important to note that natural doesn't always mean safe. Some people think that supplements—especially herbs—are safe because they are natural alternatives to the chemicals in prescription drugs. But herbs,

OTHER THERAPIES
List other therapies you use, such as physical therapy,
acupuncture or massage.

Therapy
Use
Amount
How often
Other instructions
Precautions

Therapy
Use
Amount
How often
Other instructions
Precautions

Therapy
Use
Amount
How often
Other instructions
Precautions

NOTES

too, are chemicals. And any-
thing strong enough to help also
may be strong enough to hurt.

Although many supple-
ments are touted to help
arthritis, the fact is, for most
supplements, solid scientific
evidence is not available.

That said, there are some
extracts and supplements that
have been useful in treating various types of arthritis. For example, research shows that taken
in large quantities, the omega-3
fatty acids found in oils from
certain fish modify inflammation associated with rheumatoid arthritis. Other research has
shown that oil extracted from the
borage plant has properties similar to nonsteroidal anti-inflammatory drugs (NSAIDs) without
the gastrointestinal side effects.
However, researchers have
not yet determined the effective dosages and long-term side
effects of these supplements.

For osteoarthritis, the most
popular supplements are glucosamine, which is excreted from
crab, shrimp and lobster shells,
and chondroitin sulfate, derived
from cattle trachea. Glucosamine
has been shown, in some groups
of patients, to ease OA pain.
Chondroitin is believed to draw
fluid into the joint cartilage

cartilage to help give it elasticity and slow cartilage breakdown.

For more information—including legitimate studies—on herbs and supplements, consult the Web site of the National Center for Complementary and Alternative Medicine (http://nccam.nih.gov), part of the National Institutes of Health. You can also find information about herbs and supplements used for arthritis in *Arthritis Today*'s *Supplement Guide*, online at www.arthritistoday.com.

Beyond Medication

Your doctor can prescribe medications, refer you for physical therapy or recommend weight loss or a splint, but the real responsibility for effectively managing arthritis is yours.

To take control of your arthritis, it's important to learn as much about your particular form of the disease as you can. Join an Arthritis Foundation Self-Help Course and look up information on treatment options. If you find something interesting, share it with your doctor.

Work with your doctor to find the most effective medication regimen for you—and

How You Can Use This Organizer:

Make a note of lifestyle changes you make or self-care practices you use on the pages of the Progress Report section of this organizer. Keep track of what helps and what doesn't and how you feel when you make healthy choices. Use the inside pocket to hold articles you find, and if you wish, share them with your doctor.

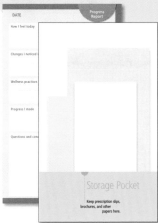

stick with it. No medication can help you if you don't take it.

At the same time, understand that medication alone isn't enough. Lifestyle factors play an important role in how you will ultimately fare with the disease. Eat healthfully, exercise regularly, lose weight if you need to or maintain a healthy weight, and avoid smoking or excessive alcohol.

Try to maintain a positive attitude. Maintain ties with friends. Continue activities you enjoy and can still do and find new, creative ways to do activities you can no longer do. Join a support group to meet others who are going through what you are and to learn how they have coped. Attend an Arthritis Foundation Exercise Class for fellowship and pain-free exercise, which has been shown to be safe and effective.

How You Can Use This Organizer:
Use the Food & Fitness Diary pages to keep track of your exercise program.

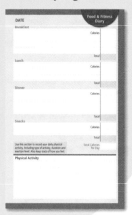

The Importance of Exercise

While exercise may be the last thing on your mind when you are tired and your joints ache, exercise may be just what you need to ease pain and improve your energy level.

Studies show that regular exercise may help reduce joint pain and stiffness, increase joint mobility and muscle strength, and improve psychological well-being. Regular exercise can also help reduce your risk of other health problems, such as heart disease or diabetes, which can accompany arthritis.

Before beginning an exercise program, it's important to speak with your doctor or physical therapist to find an appropriate exercise program for you. Ideally, your exercise program would include aerobic exercise to strengthen your heart and lungs, strengthening exercises to make your muscles stronger so they can better support your joints, and stretching exercises to keep your muscles flexible and joints moving freely. One form of exercise almost anyone with arthritis can do is water exercise. Local chapters of the Arthritis Foundation offer a warm-water Aquatic Exercise Program.

If you haven't been active for a while, start slowly and do whatever you can at first. As you become stronger and your endurance increases, you will be able to exercise longer and more strenuously.

It's also important to pay attention to your body. If a particular joint is actively inflamed, give that joint a rest, but continue to exercise. And while it's natural to experience some muscle soreness following a workout, increased joint pain may mean you're working too hard and need to scale back your exercise routine.

The Role of Diet

Although there have been many diets purported to cure arthritis, there is little evidence that any particular food or group of foods can help or hurt arthritis in everyone. But that's not to say that what you eat doesn't matter. For optimal health—whether you have arthritis or not—it's important to consume a healthful diet that is rich in vitamins and minerals and low in saturated fats and calories.

If you have an inflammatory form of arthritis, such as rheumatoid arthritis or ankylosing spondylitis, a diet high in unsaturated fats, especially fish oils, may help ease inflammation.

If you have gout, proper diet and weight loss can help keep the disease under control. Your doctor will probably advise you to limit alcohol consumption to no more than one or two drinks a day and to avoid

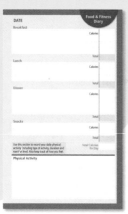
such as food as organ meats, sardines, anchovies and fish roe.

For a few people, sensitivities to certain foods may cause RA to flare. If you suspect a certain food may be aggravating your arthritis, try stopping it for a while and see if your arthritis improves. If it does, reintroduce the food to see if arthritis worsens again. If it does, avoid the food.

While eliminating a food or two probably won't hurt you, eliminating many foods or entire groups of food could make it difficult to get the nutrition you need.

When Surgery Is Needed

For most people with arthritis, a combination of medications, exercise and joint protection techniques are sufficient for managing the disease. But when joint pain is severe and unrelenting or when arthritis causes series disability, surgery may be an effective option.

There are many different types of arthritis surgeries. The best type for you, if you should need surgery, will depend on a number of factors including the particular problem and its severity, the particular joint or joints involved, your age and your treatment goals.

For example, in the early stages

of the RA, synovectomy (the surgical removal of the synovium, or lining of the joint) may be performed when one or two joints are affected by inflammation more than other joints; however, this procedure is much less common than it once was. In later stages, an arthrodesis or fusion of a joint may greatly relieve pain. An osteotomy, the correction of bone deformity by cutting and repositioning of bone such as the tibia (shin bone) or pelvis, may be used to correct joint misalignment. If severe damage to a joint (most commonly a hip or knee) has occurred, a total joint replacement or arthroplasty may dramatically relieve pain and improve a person's ability to function.

Arthritis and the Risk of Other Diseases

Unfortunately, having arthritis doesn't make you immune to other health problems. In fact, in some cases you may be more likely to have other health problems. That's because certain forms of arthritis share risk factors with other diseases. For example, obesity can increase your risk of cardiovascular disease and diabetes as well as osteoarthritis and gout. If you have rheumatoid arthritis,

you have a higher risk of other autoimmune diseases, such as type-1 diabetes and autoimmune thyroiditis, because these diseases share similar predisposing genes.

Certain medications used in arthritis treatment can also lead to other health problems. For example, disease-modifying drugs can increase your risk of infections, NSAIDs can cause gastrointestinal upset and ulcers, and corticosteroids can cause osteoporosis.

This makes it all the more important to take care of your general health if you have arthritis. Lose weight if necessary or maintain a reasonable weight, don't smoke, exercise regularly, eat a healthy diet and keep up with your doctor visits. Keeping your arthritis under control, notifying your doctor of any medication side effects and identifying and treating other problems early can help reduce your risk of further health problems and their complications. Your *Health Organizer* can help.

NOTES

Record Keeper

This section includes your health-care team and personal medical information.

How You Can Use This Section:

Use these pages to record the contact information and other pertinent information on your health-care team, hospitals and other health-care facilities, insurance providers and pharmacies.

Use the Medication sheets to record the names and dosages of medications your doctor prescribes. Make note of any possible drug side effects or interactions. Refer to these pages when speaking with your doctor or pharmacist.

Use the Laboratory Test pages to keep track of these tests and their results.

Use This Section to Record:

Health-Care Team Information
Insurance Provider Information
Hospitals And
Health-Care Facilities
Pharmacy Information
Personal Medical History
Childhood Illnesses And Diseases
Adult Illnesses And Diseases
Other Medical Conditions
Family History
Laboratory Tests
Medications: Prescription
Medications: Over-The-Counter
Other Therapies

HEALTH-CARE TEAM INFORMATION

Record the names and contact information for your
health-care team, including physicians, physical therapists,
counselors and any other specialist you visit.

Name	
Specialty	
Practice	
Address	
City/State/Zip	
Phone	After hours
Fax	Office hours
E-mail/Web site	
Nurse/Office manager	
Accepts my insurance plan?	

Name	
Specialty	
Practice	
Address	
City/State/Zip	
Phone	After hours
Fax	Office hours
E-mail/Web site	
Nurse/Office manager	
Accepts my insurance plan?	

TIP What your doctor should tell you:

- What type of arthritis or related condition you have
- What to expect
- What you can do to minimize sympoms and restore function

HEALTH-CARE TEAM INFORMATION

Record the names and contact information for your
health-care team, including physicians, physical therapists,
counselors and any other specialist you visit.

Name	
Specialty	
Practice	
Address	
City/State/Zip	
Phone	After hours
Fax	Office hours
E-mail/Web site	
Nurse/Office manager	
Accepts my insurance plan?	

Name	
Specialty	
Practice	
Address	
City/State/Zip	
Phone	After hours
Fax	Office hours
E-mail/Web site	
Nurse/Office manager	
Accepts my insurance plan?	

TIP There are more than 100 different types of arthritis
and related conditions. It is important to know which
condition you have so you can get proper treatment.

HEALTH-CARE TEAM INFORMATION

Record the names and contact information for your
health-care team, including physicians, physical therapists,
counselors and any other specialist you visit.

Name

Specialty

Practice

Address

City/State/Zip

Phone   After hours

Fax   Office hours

E-mail/Web site

Nurse/Office manager

Accepts my insurance plan?

Name

Specialty

Practice

Address

City/State/Zip

Phone   After hours

Fax   Office hours

E-mail/Web site

Nurse/Office manager

Accepts my insurance plan?

TIP An occupational therapist can show you how to reduce
strain on your joints when you perform daily activities;
a physical therapist can show you exercises to keep your
muscles strong and your joints from becoming stiff.

HEALTH-CARE TEAM INFORMATION

Record the names and contact information for your
health-care team, including physicians, physical therapists,
counselors and any other specialist you visit.

Name	
Specialty	
Practice	
Address	
City/State/Zip	
Phone	After hours
Fax	Office hours
E-mail/Web site	
Nurse/Office manager	
Accepts my insurance plan?	

Name	
Specialty	
Practice	
Address	
City/State/Zip	
Phone	After hours
Fax	Office hours
E-mail/Web site	
Nurse/Office manager	
Accepts my insurance plan?	

NOTES

HEALTH-CARE TEAM INFORMATION

Record the names and contact information for your
health-care team, including physicians, physical therapists,
counselors and any other specialist you visit.

Name

Specialty

Practice

Address

City/State/Zip

Phone   After hours

Fax   Office hours

E-mail/Web site

Nurse/Office manager

Accepts my insurance plan?

Name

Specialty

Practice

Address

City/State/Zip

Phone   After hours

Fax   Office hours

E-mail/Web site

Nurse/Office manager

Accepts my insurance plan?

NOTES

INSURANCE PROVIDER INFORMATION
List information about your health insurance policies.

Company	
Policy holder	
Policy number	
Address	
City/State/Zip	
Phone	
Fax	Contact
E-mail/Web site	
Payment Information	

Company	
Policy holder	
Policy number	
Address	
City/State/Zip	
Phone	
Fax	Contact
E-mail/Web site	
Payment Information	

TIP If you have trouble finding insurance coverage, contact your state insurance commission for names of private companies that might insure you.

INSURANCE PROVIDER INFORMATION
List information about your health insurance policies.

Company

Policy holder

Policy number

Address

City/State/Zip

Phone

Fax   Contact

E-mail/Web site

Payment Information

Company

Policy holder

Policy number

Address

City/State/Zip

Phone

Fax   Contact

E-mail/Web site

Payment Information

TIP Pre-existing condition clauses can be confusing.
Read your health insurance policy carefully so
you know what is covered and what isn't.

HOSPITALS AND
HEALTH-CARE FACILITIES
Record contact information for hospitals, clinics, rehab
centers and other facilities you use.

Name

Address

City/State/Zip

Phone

Emergency number   Fax

E-mail/Web site

Name

Address

City/State/Zip

Phone

Emergency number   Fax

E-mail/Web site

Name

Address

City/State/Zip

Phone

Emergency number   Fax

E-mail/Web site

NOTES

HOSPITALS AND HEALTH-CARE FACILITIES

Record contact information for hospitals, clinics, rehab centers and other facilities you use.

Name

Address

City/State/Zip

Phone

Emergency number   Fax

E-mail/Web site

Name

Address

City/State/Zip

Phone

Emergency number   Fax

E-mail/Web site

Name

Address

City/State/Zip

Phone

Emergency number   Fax

E-mail/Web site

NOTES

HOSPITALS AND
HEALTH-CARE FACILITIES
Record contact information for hospitals, clinics, rehab
centers and other facilities you use.

Name

Address

City/State/Zip

Phone

Emergency number   Fax

E-mail/Web site

Name

Address

City/State/Zip

Phone

Emergency number   Fax

E-mail/Web site

Name

Address

City/State/Zip

Phone

Emergency number   Fax

E-mail/Web site

NOTES

PHARMACY INFORMATION
List information about the pharmacies you use.

Name	Hours of operation
Pharmacist	Accepts my insurance?
Address	
City/State/Zip	
Phone	Fax
E-mail/Web site	

Name	Hours of operation
Pharmacist	Accepts my insurance?
Address	
City/State/Zip	
Phone	Fax
E-mail/Web site	

Name	Hours of operation
Pharmacist	Accepts my insurance?
Address	
City/State/Zip	
Phone	Fax
E-mail/Web site	

TIP Get prescriptions filled at one pharmacy if possible. That way, the records of everything you're taking will be in one place.

PHARMACY INFORMATION
List information about the pharmacies you use.

Name	Hours of operation
Pharmacist	Accepts my insurance?
Address	
City/State/Zip	
Phone	Fax
E-mail/Web site	

Name	Hours of operation
Pharmacist	Accepts my insurance?
Address	
City/State/Zip	
Phone	Fax
E-mail/Web site	

Name	Hours of operation
Pharmacist	Accepts my insurance?
Address	
City/State/Zip	
Phone	Fax
E-mail/Web site	

NOTES

PERSONAL MEDICAL HISTORY
Record information about your pesonal medical history.

Blood Type

Allergies (food, amimal hair, medications, insect bites, etc.)

Vaccinations

Type	Date

TIP If you experience difficulty breathing because of a possible allergic reaction to a medication, go to a hospital emergency room immediately or call 911. Signs of this type of medication-related allergy include rapid breathing, gasping, wheezing, fainting or rapid heartbeat.

CHILDHOOD ILLNESSES AND DISEASES

Include major illnesses you had as a child, such as measles, chicken pox, juvenile arthritis, etc.

Illness	Date

NOTES

ADULT ILLNESSES AND DISEASES
Include major illnesses you've had as an adult, such as
rheumatoid arthritis, Lyme disease, or heart disease.

Illness	Date

NOTES

OTHER MEDICAL CONDITIONS

List other conditions you have, such as high blood pressure or chronic back pain.

Condition	Date

NOTES

FAMILY HISTORY

Use this section to record information about illnesses of
close family members, such as parents or siblings.

Illness	Family Member

NOTES

SURGERIES

Use this space to record information about your surgical history.

Type	Date

TIP If you are uncertain about having surgery, get a second opinion from another doctor.

LABORATORY TESTS
Including X-Rays, bone scans, blood work

Test	Date	Result

NOTE: If you have lab tests frequently to monitor a medication you're taking, you may not need to record each test. Instead, you may want to record them periodically to show changes or trends.

TIP Lab tests help your doctor confirm a diagnosis, evaluate disease progression and check for medication side effects.

LABORATORY TESTS
Including X-Rays, bone scans, blood work

Test	Date	Result

NOTE: If you have lab tests frequently to monitor a medication you're taking, you may not need to record each test. Instead, you may want to record them periodically to show changes or trends.

NOTES

LABORATORY TESTS
Including X-Rays, bone scans, blood work

Test	Date	Result

NOTE: If you have lab tests frequently to monitor a medication you're taking, you may not need to record each test. Instead, you may want to record them periodically to show changes or trends.

NOTES

MEDICATIONS: PRESCRIPTION
List all prescription drugs you take.

Medication	Dosage
Prescribed by	
When taken	
Precautions	
Date started	Dates stopped
Possible side effects/drug interactions	

Medication	Dosage
Prescribed by	
When taken	
Precautions	
Date started	Dates stopped
Possible side effects/drug interactions	

Medication	Dosage
Prescribed by	
When taken	
Precautions	
Date started	Dates stopped
Possible side effects/drug interactions	

TIP To avoid confusion, keep your medications in properly labeled containers.

MEDICATIONS: PRESCRIPTION
List all prescription drugs you take.

Medication	Dosage
Prescribed by	
When taken	
Precautions	
Date started	Dates stopped
Possible side effects/drug interactions	

Medication	Dosage
Prescribed by	
When taken	
Precautions	
Date started	Dates stopped
Possible side effects/drug interactions	

Medication	Dosage
Prescribed by	
When taken	
Precautions	
Date started	Dates stopped
Possible side effects/drug interactions	

NOTES

MEDICATIONS: PRESCRIPTION
List all prescription drugs you take.

Medication	Dosage
Prescribed by	
When taken	
Precautions	
Date started	Dates stopped
Possible side effects/drug interactions	

Medication	Dosage
Prescribed by	
When taken	
Precautions	
Date started	Dates stopped
Possible side effects/drug interactions	

Medication	Dosage
Prescribed by	
When taken	
Precautions	
Date started	Dates stopped
Possible side effects/drug interactions	

NOTES

MEDICATIONS: PRESCRIPTION
List all prescription drugs you take.

Medication	Dosage

Prescribed by

When taken

Precautions

Date started	Dates stopped

Possible side effects/drug interactions

Medication	Dosage

Prescribed by

When taken

Precautions

Date started	Dates stopped

Possible side effects/drug interactions

Medication	Dosage

Prescribed by

When taken

Precautions

Date started	Dates stopped

Possible side effects/drug interactions

NOTES

MEDICATIONS: OVER-THE-COUNTER

List all over-the-counter drugs you take, such as pain
relievers or antacids.

Medication

Used for

Amount taken

How often

Precautions

Possible side effects/drug interactions

Medication

Used for

Amount taken

How often

Precautions

Possible side effects/drug interactions

Medication

Used for

Amount taken

How often

Precautions

Possible side effects/drug interactions

TIP Over-the-counter medications are approved for lower doses than
prescription products. Do not take more than the amount listed
on the bottle without consulting your doctor.

MEDICATIONS: OVER-THE-COUNTER

List all over-the-counter drugs you take, such as pain relievers or antacids.

Record Keeper

Medication

Used for

Amount taken

How often

Precautions

Possible side effects/drug interactions

Medication

Used for

Amount taken

How often

Precautions

Possible side effects/drug interactions

Medication

Used for

Amount taken

How often

Precautions

Possible side effects/drug interactions

NOTES

MEDICATIONS: OVER-THE-COUNTER

List all over-the-counter drugs you take, such as pain relievers or antacids.

Medication

Used for

Amount taken

How often

Precautions

Possible side effects/drug interactions

Medication

Used for

Amount taken

How often

Precautions

Possible side effects/drug interactions

Medication

Used for

Amount taken

How often

Precautions

Possible side effects/drug interactions

NOTES

MEDICATIONS: OVER-THE-COUNTER
List all over-the-counter drugs you take, such as pain relievers or antacids.

Medication

Used for

Amount taken

How often

Precautions

Possible side effects/drug interactions

Medication

Used for

Amount taken

How often

Precautions

Possible side effects/drug interactions

Medication

Used for

Amount taken

How often

Precautions

Possible side effects/drug interactions

NOTES

OTHER THERAPIES
List other therapies you use, such as physical therapy,
acupuncture or massage.

Therapy

Use

Amount

How often

Other instructions

Precautions

Therapy

Use

Amount

How often

Other instructions

Precautions

Therapy

Use

Amount

How often

Other instructions

Precautions

TIP Before you try a therapy or treatment, check your insurance
policy carefully to find out exactly what is covered.

OTHER THERAPIES

List other therapies you use, such as physical therapy,
acupuncture or massage.

Therapy

Use

Amount

How often

Other instructions

Precautions

Therapy

Use

Amount

How often

Other instructions

Precautions

Therapy

Use

Amount

How often

Other instructions

Precautions

NOTES

OTHER THERAPIES
List other therapies you use, such as physical therapy,
acupuncture or massage.

Therapy

Use

Amount

How often

Other instructions

Precautions

Therapy

Use

Amount

How often

Other instructions

Precautions

Therapy

Use

Amount

How often

Other instructions

Precautions

NOTES

Progress Report

In this section, record trends and progress in your health.

How You Can Use This Section:

Use the Progress Report pages to keep track of your health and note changes – good or bad – in your health.

Use the Progress Report to note any questions about medications, test results and symptoms you'd like to bring up at your next office visit.

Also make a note of lifestyle changes you make or self-care practices you use. Keep track of what helps and what doesn't and how you feel when you make healthy choices.

Use This Section to Record:

How You Feel Each Day
Changes In Health
Wellness Practices
Progress
Questions And Concerns

How I feel today

Changes I noticed in my health

Wellness practices I followed (such as exercise, relaxation, joint protection)

Progress I made

Questions and concerns to discuss with my doctor or other health-care provider

DATE

How I feel today

Changes I noticed in my health

Wellness practices I followed (such as exercise, relaxation, joint protection)

Progress I made

Questions and concerns to discuss with my doctor or other health-care provider

DATE

How I feel today

Changes I noticed in my health

Wellness practices I followed (such as exercise, relaxation, joint protection)

Progress I made

Questions and concerns to discuss with my doctor or other health-care provider

How I feel today

Changes I noticed in my health

Wellness practices I followed (such as exercise, relaxation, joint protection)

Progress I made

Questions and concerns to discuss with my doctor or other health-care provider

How I feel today

Changes I noticed in my health

Wellness practices I followed (such as exercise, relaxation, joint protection)

Progress I made

Questions and concerns to discuss with my doctor or other health-care provider

How I feel today

Changes I noticed in my health

Wellness practices I followed (such as exercise, relaxation, joint protection)

Progress I made

Questions and concerns to discuss with my doctor or other health-care provider

DATE

How I feel today

Changes I noticed in my health

Wellness practices I followed (such as exercise, relaxation, joint protection)

Progress I made

Questions and concerns to discuss with my doctor or other health-care provider

DATE

How I feel today

Changes I noticed in my health

Wellness practices I followed (such as exercise, relaxation, joint protection)

Progress I made

Questions and concerns to discuss with my doctor or other health-care provider

NOTES

DATE

How I feel today

Changes I noticed in my health

Wellness practices I followed (such as exercise, relaxation, joint protection)

Progress I made

Questions and concerns to discuss with my doctor or other health-care provider

NOTES

DATE

How I feel today

Changes I noticed in my health

Wellness practices I followed (such as exercise, relaxation, joint protection)

Progress I made

Questions and concerns to discuss with my doctor or other health-care provider

DATE

How I feel today

Changes I noticed in my health

Wellness practices I followed (such as exercise, relaxation, joint protection)

Progress I made

Questions and concerns to discuss with my doctor or other health-care provider

DATE

How I feel today

Changes I noticed in my health

Wellness practices I followed (such as exercise, relaxation, joint protection)

Progress I made

Questions and concerns to discuss with my doctor or other health-care provider

How I feel today

Changes I noticed in my health

Wellness practices I followed (such as exercise, relaxation, joint protection)

Progress I made

Questions and concerns to discuss with my doctor or other health-care provider

DATE

How I feel today

Changes I noticed in my health

Wellness practices I followed (such as exercise, relaxation, joint protection)

Progress I made

Questions and concerns to discuss with my doctor or other health-care provider

How I feel today

Changes I noticed in my health

Wellness practices I followed (such as exercise, relaxation, joint protection)

Progress I made

Questions and concerns to discuss with my doctor or other health-care provider

DATE

How I feel today

Changes I noticed in my health

Wellness practices I followed (such as exercise, relaxation, joint protection)

Progress I made

Questions and concerns to discuss with my doctor or other health-care provider

DATE

How I feel today

Changes I noticed in my health

Wellness practices I followed (such as exercise, relaxation, joint protection)

Progress I made

Questions and concerns to discuss with my doctor or other health-care provider

NOTES

How I feel today

Changes I noticed in my health

Wellness practices I followed (such as exercise, relaxation, joint protection)

Progress I made

Questions and concerns to discuss with my doctor or other health-care provider

DATE

How I feel today

Changes I noticed in my health

Wellness practices I followed (such as exercise, relaxation, joint protection)

Progress I made

Questions and concerns to discuss with my doctor or other health-care provider

DATE

How I feel today

Changes I noticed in my health

Wellness practices I followed (such as exercise, relaxation, joint protection)

Progress I made

Questions and concerns to discuss with my doctor or other health-care provider

How I feel today

Changes I noticed in my health

Wellness practices I followed (such as exercise, relaxation, joint protection)

Progress I made

Questions and concerns to discuss with my doctor or other health-care provider

How I feel today

Changes I noticed in my health

Wellness practices I followed (such as exercise, relaxation, joint protection)

Progress I made

Questions and concerns to discuss with my doctor or other health-care provider

How I feel today

Changes I noticed in my health

Wellness practices I followed (such as exercise, relaxation, joint protection)

Progress I made

Questions and concerns to discuss with my doctor or other health-care provider

How I feel today

Changes I noticed in my health

Wellness practices I followed (such as exercise, relaxation, joint protection)

Progress I made

Questions and concerns to discuss with my doctor or other health-care provider

How I feel today

Changes I noticed in my health

Wellness practices I followed (such as exercise, relaxation, joint protection)

Progress I made

Questions and concerns to discuss with my doctor or other health-care provider

DATE

How I feel today

Changes I noticed in my health

Wellness practices I followed (such as exercise, relaxation, joint protection)

Progress I made

Questions and concerns to discuss with my doctor or other health-care provider

How I feel today

Changes I noticed in my health

Wellness practices I followed (such as exercise, relaxation, joint protection)

Progress I made

Questions and concerns to discuss with my doctor or other health-care provider

DATE

How I feel today

Changes I noticed in my health

Wellness practices I followed (such as exercise, relaxation, joint protection)

Progress I made

Questions and concerns to discuss with my doctor or other health-care provider

DATE

Progress Report

How I feel today

Changes I noticed in my health

Wellness practices I followed (such as exercise, relaxation, joint protection)

Progress I made

Questions and concerns to discuss with my doctor or other health-care provider

How I feel today

Changes I noticed in my health

Wellness practices I followed (such as exercise, relaxation, joint protection)

Progress I made

Questions and concerns to discuss with my doctor or other health-care provider

How I feel today

Changes I noticed in my health

Wellness practices I followed (such as exercise, relaxation, joint protection)

Progress I made

Questions and concerns to discuss with my doctor or other health-care provider

How I feel today

Changes I noticed in my health

Wellness practices I followed (such as exercise, relaxation, joint protection)

Progress I made

Questions and concerns to discuss with my doctor or other health-care provider

Food & Fitness Diary

In this section, keep track of your diet and exercise.

How You Can Use This Section:

Use the Food & Fitness Diary pages to keep track of your
eating habits and your daily activity.

The Food & Fitness Diary pages are a good place to note
any changes you make in your diet. Looking back at
the pages over time can help you identify possible links
between symptoms and certain foods.

Record your physical activity for each day, and note how
you feel when you exercise.

Use This Section to Record:

What You Eat
Daily Calorie Intake
Physical Activity
Type of Exercise
Duration of Activity
Exertion Level

DATE

Breakfast

	Calories
	Total

Lunch

	Calories
	Total

Dinner

	Calories
	Total

Snacks

	Calories
	Total

Use this section to record your daily physical activity, including type of activity, duration and exertion level. Also keep track of how you feel.

Total Calories for Day

Physical Activity

DATE

Breakfast

	Calories
Total	

Lunch

	Calories
Total	

Dinner

	Calories
Total	

Snacks

	Calories
Total	

Use this section to record your daily physical activity, including type of activity, duration and exertion level. Also keep track of how you feel.

Total Calories for Day

Physical Activity

DATE

Breakfast

Calories

Total

Lunch

Calories

Total

Dinner

Calories

Total

Snacks

Calories

Total

Use this section to record your daily physical activity, including type of activity, duration and exertion level. Also keep track of how you feel.

Total Calories for Day

Physical Activity

DATE

Breakfast

	Calories
Total	

Lunch

	Calories
Total	

Dinner

	Calories
Total	

Snacks

	Calories
Total	

Use this section to record your daily physical activity, including type of activity, duration and exertion level. Also keep track of how you feel.

Total Calories for Day

Physical Activity

DATE

Breakfast

	Calories
	Total

Lunch

	Calories
	Total

Dinner

	Calories
	Total

Snacks

	Calories
	Total

Use this section to record your daily physical activity, including type of activity, duration and exertion level. Also keep track of how you feel.

Total Calories for Day

Physical Activity

DATE

Breakfast

	Calories
Total	

Lunch

	Calories
Total	

Dinner

	Calories
Total	

Snacks

	Calories
Total	

Use this section to record your daily physical activity, including type of activity, duration and exertion level. Also keep track of how you feel.

Total Calories for Day

Physical Activity

DATE

Breakfast

Calories

Total

Lunch

Calories

Total

Dinner

Calories

Total

Snacks

Calories

Total

Use this section to record your daily physical activity, including type of activity, duration and exertion level. Also keep track of how you feel.

Total Calories for Day

Physical Activity

DATE

Breakfast

	Calories	
	Total	

Lunch

	Calories	
	Total	

Dinner

	Calories	
	Total	

Snacks

	Calories	
	Total	

Use this section to record your daily physical activity, including type of activity, duration and exertion level. Also keep track of how you feel.

Total Calories for Day

Physical Activity

DATE

Breakfast

Calories

Total

Lunch

Calories

Total

Dinner

Calories

Total

Snacks

Calories

Total

Use this section to record your daily physical activity, including type of activity, duration and exertion level. Also keep track of how you feel.

Total Calories for Day

Physical Activity

DATE

Breakfast

	Calories
Total	

Lunch

	Calories
Total	

Dinner

	Calories
Total	

Snacks

	Calories
Total	

Use this section to record your daily physical activity, including type of activity, duration and exertion level. Also keep track of how you feel.

Total Calories for Day

Physical Activity

DATE

Breakfast

	Calories	
	Total	

Lunch

	Calories	
	Total	

Dinner

	Calories	
	Total	

Snacks

	Calories	
	Total	

Use this section to record your daily physical activity, including type of activity, duration and exertion level. Also keep track of how you feel.

Total Calories for Day

Physical Activity

DATE

Breakfast

	Calories	
	Total	

Lunch

	Calories	
	Total	

Dinner

	Calories	
	Total	

Snacks

	Calories	
	Total	

Use this section to record your daily physical activity, including type of activity, duration and exertion level. Also keep track of how you feel.

Total Calories for Day	

Physical Activity

DATE

Breakfast

	Calories	
	Total	

Lunch

	Calories	
	Total	

Dinner

	Calories	
	Total	

Snacks

	Calories	
	Total	

Use this section to record your daily physical activity, including type of activity, duration and exertion level. Also keep track of how you feel.

Total Calories for Day

Physical Activity

DATE

Breakfast

	Calories	
	Total	

Lunch

	Calories	
	Total	

Dinner

	Calories	
	Total	

Snacks

	Calories	
	Total	

Use this section to record your daily physical activity, including type of activity, duration and exertion level. Also keep track of how you feel.

Total Calories for Day

Physical Activity

DATE

Breakfast

	Calories
Total	

Lunch

	Calories
Total	

Dinner

	Calories
Total	

Snacks

	Calories
Total	

Use this section to record your daily physical activity, including type of activity, duration and exertion level. Also keep track of how you feel.

Total Calories for Day

Physical Activity

DATE

Breakfast

	Calories	
	Total	

Lunch

	Calories	
	Total	

Dinner

	Calories	
	Total	

Snacks

	Calories	
	Total	

Use this section to record your daily physical activity, including type of activity, duration and exertion level. Also keep track of how you feel.

Total Calories for Day

Physical Activity

DATE

Breakfast

Calories

Total

Lunch

Calories

Total

Dinner

Calories

Total

Snacks

Calories

Total

Use this section to record your daily physical activity, including type of activity, duration and exertion level. Also keep track of how you feel.

Total Calories
for Day

Physical Activity

DATE

Breakfast

	Calories
Total	

Lunch

	Calories
Total	

Dinner

	Calories
Total	

Snacks

	Calories
Total	

Use this section to record your daily physical activity, including type of activity, duration and exertion level. Also keep track of how you feel.

Total Calories for Day

Physical Activity

DATE

Breakfast

	Calories
Total	

Lunch

	Calories
Total	

Dinner

	Calories
Total	

Snacks

	Calories
Total	

Use this section to record your daily physical activity, including type of activity, duration and exertion level. Also keep track of how you feel.

Total Calories for Day

Physical Activity

DATE

Breakfast

	Calories
Total	

Lunch

	Calories
Total	

Dinner

	Calories
Total	

Snacks

	Calories
Total	

Use this section to record your daily physical activity, including type of activity, duration and exertion level. Also keep track of how you feel.

Total Calories for Day

Physical Activity

DATE

Breakfast

	Calories
Total	

Lunch

	Calories
Total	

Dinner

	Calories
Total	

Snacks

	Calories
Total	

Use this section to record your daily physical activity, including type of activity, duration and exertion level. Also keep track of how you feel.

Total Calories for Day

Physical Activity

DATE

Breakfast

	Calories
Total	

Lunch

	Calories
Total	

Dinner

	Calories
Total	

Snacks

	Calories
Total	

Use this section to record your daily physical activity, including type of activity, duration and exertion level. Also keep track of how you feel.

Total Calories for Day

Physical Activity

DATE

Breakfast

	Calories	
	Total	

Lunch

	Calories	
	Total	

Dinner

	Calories	
	Total	

Snacks

	Calories	
	Total	

Use this section to record your daily physical activity, including type of activity, duration and exertion level. Also keep track of how you feel.

Total Calories for Day

Physical Activity

DATE

Breakfast

	Calories
Total	

Lunch

	Calories
Total	

Dinner

	Calories
Total	

Snacks

	Calories
Total	

Use this section to record your daily physical activity, including type of activity, duration and exertion level. Also keep track of how you feel.

Total Calories for Day

Physical Activity

DATE

Breakfast

	Calories	
	Total	

Lunch

	Calories	
	Total	

Dinner

	Calories	
	Total	

Snacks

	Calories	
	Total	

Use this section to record your daily physical activity, including type of activity, duration and exertion level. Also keep track of how you feel.

Total Calories for Day

Physical Activity

DATE

Breakfast

	Calories
Total	

Lunch

	Calories
Total	

Dinner

	Calories
Total	

Snacks

	Calories
Total	

Use this section to record your daily physical activity, including type of activity, duration and exertion level. Also keep track of how you feel.

Total Calories for Day

Physical Activity

DATE

Breakfast

	Calories
	Total

Lunch

	Calories
	Total

Dinner

	Calories
	Total

Snacks

	Calories
	Total

Use this section to record your daily physical activity, including type of activity, duration and exertion level. Also keep track of how you feel.

Total Calories for Day

Physical Activity

DATE

Breakfast

	Calories
Total	

Lunch

	Calories
Total	

Dinner

	Calories
Total	

Snacks

	Calories
Total	

Use this section to record your daily physical activity, including type of activity, duration and exertion level. Also keep track of how you feel.

Total Calories for Day	

Physical Activity

DATE

Breakfast

Calories

Total

Lunch

Calories

Total

Dinner

Calories

Total

Snacks

Calories

Total

Use this section to record your daily physical activity, including type of activity, duration and exertion level. Also keep track of how you feel.

Total Calories for Day

Physical Activity

DATE

Breakfast

	Calories
Total	

Lunch

	Calories
Total	

Dinner

	Calories
Total	

Snacks

	Calories
Total	

Use this section to record your daily physical activity, including type of activity, duration and exertion level. Also keep track of how you feel.

Total Calories for Day

Physical Activity

DATE

Breakfast

	Calories	
	Total	

Lunch

	Calories	
	Total	

Dinner

	Calories	
	Total	

Snacks

	Calories	
	Total	

Use this section to record your daily physical activity, including type of activity, duration and exertion level. Also keep track of how you feel.

Total Calories for Day

Physical Activity

DATE

Breakfast

	Calories
Total	

Lunch

	Calories
Total	

Dinner

	Calories
Total	

Snacks

	Calories
Total	

Use this section to record your daily physical activity, including type of activity, duration and exertion level. Also keep track of how you feel.

Total Calories for Day

Physical Activity

DATE

Breakfast

	Calories
	Total

Lunch

	Calories
	Total

Dinner

	Calories
	Total

Snacks

	Calories
	Total

Use this section to record your daily physical activity, including type of activity, duration and exertion level. Also keep track of how you feel.

Total Calories for Day

Physical Activity

DATE

Breakfast

	Calories	
	Total	

Lunch

	Calories	
	Total	

Dinner

	Calories	
	Total	

Snacks

	Calories	
	Total	

Use this section to record your daily physical activity, including type of activity, duration and exertion level. Also keep track of how you feel.

Total Calories for Day	

Physical Activity

DATE

Breakfast

	Calories
	Total

Lunch

	Calories
	Total

Dinner

	Calories
	Total

Snacks

	Calories
	Total

Use this section to record your daily physical activity, including type of activity, duration and exertion level. Also keep track of how you feel.

Total Calories for Day

Physical Activity

DATE

Breakfast

	Calories
Total	

Lunch

	Calories
Total	

Dinner

	Calories
Total	

Snacks

	Calories
Total	

Use this section to record your daily physical activity, including type of activity, duration and exertion level. Also keep track of how you feel.

Total Calories for Day	

Physical Activity

DATE

Breakfast

	Calories
	Total

Lunch

	Calories
	Total

Dinner

	Calories
	Total

Snacks

	Calories
	Total

Use this section to record your daily physical activity, including type of activity, duration and exertion level. Also keep track of how you feel.

Total Calories for Day

Physical Activity

DATE

Breakfast

	Calories
Total	

Lunch

	Calories
Total	

Dinner

	Calories
Total	

Snacks

	Calories
Total	

Use this section to record your daily physical activity, including type of activity, duration and exertion level. Also keep track of how you feel.

Total Calories for Day

Physical Activity

DATE

Breakfast

	Calories
	Total

Lunch

	Calories
	Total

Dinner

	Calories
	Total

Snacks

	Calories
	Total

Use this section to record your daily physical activity, including type of activity, duration and exertion level. Also keep track of how you feel.

Total Calories for Day

Physical Activity

DATE

Breakfast

	Calories
Total	

Lunch

	Calories
Total	

Dinner

	Calories
Total	

Snacks

	Calories
Total	

Use this section to record your daily physical activity, including type of activity, duration and exertion level. Also keep track of how you feel.

Total Calories for Day

Physical Activity

DATE

Breakfast

	Calories
	Total

Lunch

	Calories
	Total

Dinner

	Calories
	Total

Snacks

	Calories
	Total

Use this section to record your daily physical activity, including type of activity, duration and exertion level. Also keep track of how you feel.

Total Calories for Day

Physical Activity

DATE

Breakfast

	Calories
Total	

Lunch

	Calories
Total	

Dinner

	Calories
Total	

Snacks

	Calories
Total	

Use this section to record your daily physical activity, including type of activity, duration and exertion level. Also keep track of how you feel.

Total Calories for Day

Physical Activity

DATE

Breakfast

	Calories
Total	

Lunch

	Calories
Total	

Dinner

	Calories
Total	

Snacks

	Calories
Total	

Use this section to record your daily physical activity, including type of activity, duration and exertion level. Also keep track of how you feel.

Total Calories for Day	

Physical Activity

DATE

Breakfast

	Calories	
	Total	

Lunch

	Calories	
	Total	

Dinner

	Calories	
	Total	

Snacks

	Calories	
	Total	

Use this section to record your daily physical activity, including type of activity, duration and exertion level. Also keep track of how you feel.

	Total Calories for Day	

Physical Activity

DATE

Breakfast

	Calories
	Total

Lunch

	Calories
	Total

Dinner

	Calories
	Total

Snacks

	Calories
	Total

Use this section to record your daily physical activity, including type of activity, duration and exertion level. Also keep track of how you feel.

Total Calories for Day

Physical Activity

DATE

Breakfast

	Calories
Total	

Lunch

	Calories
Total	

Dinner

	Calories
Total	

Snacks

	Calories
Total	

Use this section to record your daily physical activity, including type of activity, duration and exertion level. Also keep track of how you feel.

Total Calories for Day

Physical Activity

DATE

Breakfast

	Calories
Total	

Lunch

	Calories
Total	

Dinner

	Calories
Total	

Snacks

	Calories
Total	

Use this section to record your daily physical activity, including type of activity, duration and exertion level. Also keep track of how you feel.

Total Calories for Day

Physical Activity

DATE

Breakfast

	Calories
Total	

Lunch

	Calories
Total	

Dinner

	Calories
Total	

Snacks

	Calories
Total	

Use this section to record your daily physical activity, including type of activity, duration and exertion level. Also keep track of how you feel.

	Total Calories for Day

Physical Activity

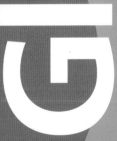

Glossary

This section contains definitions of words that may be helpful in understanding your health.

How You Can Use This Section:

The Glossary section contains definitions of almost 200 terms commonly used in the diagnosis and treatment of arthritis. Knowing these words will help you feel more at ease discussing your condition.

Use This Section to Record:

Unknown Medical Terms to Look Up
Additional Terms and Definitions
Notes

acupressure Eastern medicine technique in which pressure is applied to specific sites along energy pathways called meridians.

acupuncture Eastern medicine technique in which needles are used to puncture the body at specific sites along energy pathways called meridians.

acute illness Disease that can be severe, but of short duration, unlike chronic illness.

acute pain See pain.

adrenal glands Glands located near the kidneys. These glands secrete a variety of hormones, including glucocorticoids.

adrenaline A hormone that increases the heart and respiration rate when we feel frightened, threatened or angry, preparing us to flee to safety, or stand and fight.

aerobic An activity designed to increase oxygen consumption by the body, such as aerobic exercise or aerobic breathing.

alternative therapy Any practice or substance outside the realm of conventional medicine.

American College of Rheumatology (ACR) An organization that provides a professional, educational, and research forum for rheumatologists across the country. Its functions include helping determine what symptoms and signs define rheumatic disease diagnoses and what the appropriate treatments are for those diagnoses.

analgesic Drugs used to help relieve pain.

anemia A condition marked by a reduction in the number of red blood cells, amount of hemoglobin in the blood, or total blood volume.

anemia, iron deficiency Anemia resulting from a greater demand on the stored iron than can be supplied.

anemia, pernicious Anemia resulting from a lack of vitamin B12; it is associated with absence of hydrochloric acid in the stomach.

anesthesia Chemicals that induce a partial or complete loss of sensation. Used to perform surgery and other medical procedures.

anesthesiologist A physician specializing in the administration of anesthesia.

ankylosing spondylitis Form of arthritis that primarily affects the joints and ligaments of the spine, marked by pain and stiffness. Can result in fusion of joints and bones, leading to rigidity.

antibody A specialized protein that neutralizes antigens, or foreign substances, in the body.

antigen A foreign substance that begins an immune reaction in the body.

antinuclear antibody test Test used to detect presence of abnormal antibodies.

arthritis From the Greek word "arth" meaning "joint," and the suffix "itis" meaning "inflammation." It generally means involvement of a joint from any cause, such as infection, trauma or inflammation.

arthrodesis A surgical procedure involving the fusing of two bones.

arthroplasty A surgical procedure to replace a joint with an artificial one.

arthroscopic surgery A type of surgery using an instrument, called an arthroscope, consisting of a thin tube with a light at one end, inserted into the body through a small incision, and connected to a closed-circuit television.

aspiration The removal of a substance by suction. Technique used to remove fluid from an inflamed joint, both to relieve pressure and to examine the fluid.

autoantibody antibodies acting against the body's own tissues.

autoimmune disorder An illness in which the body's immune system mistakenly attacks and damages tissues of the body. There are many types of autoimmune disorders, including arthritis and the rheumatic diseases.

biologic response modifiers Drugs that target the specific components of the immune system that contribute to disease. Includes etanercept and infliximab.

biomedical model Traditional model of medical care, based on the principle of identifying a single cause and cure for each disease.

biopsychosocial model More recent model of medical care, in which a patient's self-management plays a part in the treatment of chronic disease, and biological, psychological and socioeconomic factors are considered influential to the disease's outcome.

body mechanics The structures and methods with which your body moves and performs physical tasks.

bone densitometry Imaging study used to measure bone density, particularly in diagnosing osteoporosis.

bunion Inflammation, enlargement and malalignment of the joint of the great toe.

bursa A small sac located between a tendon and a bone. The bursae (plural for bursa) reduce friction and provide lubrication. See also bursitis.

bursitis Inflammation of a bursa (see bursa above), which can occur when the joint has been overused or when the joint has become deformed by arthritis. Bursitis makes it painful to move or put pressure on the affected joint.

C-reactive protein Protein that indicates inflammation when found in elevated levels in the body.

capsaicin A pain-killing chemical contained in some hot peppers, which gives the peppers their "burn." Available in nonprescription creams that can be rubbed on the skin over a joint to relieve pain.

cartilage A firm, smooth, rubbery substance that provides a gliding surface for joint motion, and prevents bone-on-bone contact.

chiropodist a doctor with particular training in the care of the feet. Also called podiatrist.

chronic illness Disease of a long duration, such as rheumatoid arthritis.

chronic pain Pain that is constant or persists over a long period , perhaps throughout life. See pain.

circadian rhythm The daily, monthly and seasonal schedules of essential biologic tasks, such as eating, digesting, eliminating, growing and resting. Disruption of these rhythms – when you travel rapidly across time zones (promoting "jet lag"), for example – has a negative and sometimes profound impact on performance and mood.

complementary therapy Any practice or substance used in conjunction with traditional treatment.

control group A group of people used as a standard for comparison in scientific studies.

cool-down exercises A series of physical activities that allow your heart and respiration rates to return to normal after being elevated by exercise.

corticosteroids see glucocorticoids.

cortisone A hormone produced by the cortex of the adrenal gland. Cortisone has potent anti-inflammatory effects but can also have side effects. See also glucocorticoids.

Cox-2 inhibitors Drugs that inhibit inflammation and are designed to have fewer gastrointestinal side effects than traditional NSAIDs. Includes celecoxib.

cytokines Chemicals involved in the inflammatory response.

cytotoxic drugs Chemicals that destroy cells or prevent their multiplication.

deconditioning Loss of muscle mass and strength because of inactivity. See also reconditioning.

deep breathing Drawing air into the lungs, filling them as much as possible, and then exhaling slowly. Performing this type of rhythmic breathing for a few minutes increases the amount of oxygen refreshing your brain and produces relaxation and readiness for mental tasks.

depression A state of mind characterized by gloominess, dejection or sadness.

depression, clinical A recognized mental illness in which the feelings of depression are severe, prolonged and hamper your ability to function normally.

dermatomyositis See polymyositis.

disease Sickness. Some physicians use this term only for conditions in which a structural or functional change in tissues or organs has been identified.

disorder An ailment; an abnormal health condition.

DMARDs Disease modifying antirheumatic drugs, used to slow or stop the progression of inflammatory joint disease. Includes methotrexate.

dose-pack A package of glucocorticoid drugs with a tapered daily dosage.

double-blind studies A method used in scientific studies to compare one intervention (such as a new medication) with other interventions, or no intervention. In this method, the study participants and the persons evaluating the interventions are "blinded" – that is, they aren't told who is getting the intervention being tested – so their responses will not be influenced by their opinions or expectations of the intervention.

endorphins Natural painkillers produced by the human nervous system that have qualities similar to opiate drugs. Endorphins are released during exercise and when we laugh.

endurance exercises Exercises such as swimming, walking and cycling that use the large muscles of the body and are dependent on increasing the amount of oxygen that reaches the muscles. These exercises strengthen muscles and increase and maintain physical fitness.

enthesis The place where the tendon inserts into the bone.

ergonomics The study of human capabilities and limitations in relation to the work system, machine or task, as well as the study of the physical, psychological and social environment of the worker. Also known as "human engineering."

erosions Small holes near the ends of bones.

erythrocyte sedimentation rate A test measuring how fast red blood cells (erythrocytes) fall to the bottom of a test tube, indicating level of inflammation. Often called ESR or "sed rate."

fatigue A general worn-down feeling of no energy. Fatigue can be caused by excessive physical, mental or emotional exertion, by lack of sleep, and by inflammation or disease.

Felty's syndrome Form of rheumatoid arthritis marked by an enlargement of the spleen and a reduced number of white blood cells.

fibromyalgia A noninfectious rheumatic condition affecting the body's soft tissue. Characterized by muscle pain, fatigue and nonrestorative sleep, fibromyalgia produces no abnormal X-ray or laboratory findings. It is often associated with headaches and irritable bowel syndrome.

flare A term used to describe times when the disease or condition is at its worst.

flexibility exercises Muscle stretches and other activities designed to maintain flexibility and to prevent stiffness or shortening of ligaments and tendons.

Food Labeling Act Recent legal decree of the U.S. government mandating the type of information that must be given on food labels regarding nutritional content. This Act ensures that consumers will have easy-to-read fat, protein, fiber, carbohydrate and calorie content information, and more.

gate theory A theory of how pain signals travel to the brain. According to this theory, pain signals must pass a "pain gate" that can be opened or closed by various positive (e.g., feelings of happiness) or negative (e.g., feelings of sadness) factors.

genetic predisposition Susceptibility to a specific disease or illness caused by certain inherited characteristics.

glucocorticoids A group of hormones including cortisol produced by the adrenal glands. They can also be synthetically produced (that is, made in a laboratory) and have powerful anti-inflammatory affects. These are sometimes called corticosteroids or steroids, but they are not the same as the dangerous performance-enhancing drugs that some athletes use to promote strength and endurance.

gout Disease that occurs due to an excess of uric acid in the blood, causing crystals to deposit in the joint, leading to pain and inflammation.

grief Feelings of loss; acute sorrow.

guided imagery A method of

managing pain and stress. Following the voice of a "guide," an audiotape or videotape, or one's own internal voice, attention is focused on a series of images that lead one's mind away from the stressor or pain.

H2 blockers Compounds that act by blocking receptors in the stomach that lead to the production of acid.

hammer toes A specific type of joint malalignment of the toes seen in rheumatoid arthritis.

helplessness The concept of not feeling in control of your life or your health.

hematocrit The percentage of red blood cells found in blood.

hemoglobin The protein in red blood cells that carries oxygen from the lungs to the tissues.

hormones Concentrated chemical substances produced in the glands or organs that have specific – and usually multiple – regulating effects on the body.

illness Poor health; sickness.

immune response Activation of the body's immune system.

immune system Your body's complex biochemical system for defending itself against bacteria, viruses, wounds and other injuries. Among the many components of the system are a variety of cells (such as T cells), organs (such as the lymph glands) and chemicals (such as histamine and prostaglandins).

inflammation A response to injury or infection that involves a sequence of biochemical reactions. Inflammation can be generalized, causing fatigue, fever, and pain or tenderness all over the body.

It can also be localized, for example, in joints, where it causes swelling and pain. In rheumatoid arthritis, inflammation is not caused by injury or infection, but is part of an autoimmune reaction.

internist A physician who specializes in internal medicine; sometimes called a primary-care physician.

isometric exercises Exercises that build the muscles around joints by tightening the muscles without moving the joints.

isotonic exercises Exercises that strengthen muscles by moving the joints.

joint The place or part where one bone connects to another.

joint count An examination done by a doctor to determine the number of joints that are affected by arthritis.

joint malalignment When joints are not aligned properly, due to joint damage.

joint replacement surgery Also known as arthroplasty, a surgical procedure involving the reconstruction or replacement (with a man-made component) of a joint.

ligament Flexible band of fibrous tissue that connects bones to one another.

locus The site of a gene on a chromosome.

lupus (systemic lupus erythematosus) The term used to describe an inflammatory connective tissue autoimmune disease that can involve the skin, joints, kidneys, blood and other organs. Associated with antinuclear antibodies.

malalignment, joint When

joints are not aligned properly, due to joint damage.

massage A technique of applying pressure, friction or vibration to the muscles, by hand or using a massage appliance, to stimulate circulation and produce relaxation and pain relief.

massage therapist One who has completed a program of study and is licensed to perform massage.

meditation A sustained period of deep inward thought, reflection and openness to inspiration.

meridians Energy pathways used in Eastern medicine, but that have no Western medicine counterparts.

morbidity (rate) The frequency or proportion of people with a particular diagnosis or disability in a given population.

MRI Magnetic Resonance Imaging test, a scan used as a diagnostic aid.

muscle Tissue that moves organs or parts of the body.

myalgia Pain of the muscles.

narcotic A class of drug that reduces pain by blocking signals traveling from the central nervous system to the brain. Although narcotics have the potential to be addictive and are sometimes abused , they can be used safely under skilled medical supervision for effective pain relief.

NSAID (nonsteroidal anti-inflammatory drug) A type of drug that does not contain steroids but is used to relieve pain and reduce inflammation.

nurse A person who has received education and training in health care, particularly patient care.

nurse practitioner A registered nurse with advanced training and emphasis in primary care.

objective Capable of being observed or measured; for example, infection can be objectively observed by the presence of bacteria in a blood test or culture test. See also subjective.

occupational therapist A health professional who teaches patients to reduce strain on joints while doing everyday activities.

orthopaedic surgeon A surgeon who specializes in diseases of the bone.

orthopaedist A physician who specializes in diseases of the bone.

osteoarthritis A disease causing cartilage breakdown in certain joints (spine, hands, hips, knees) resulting in pain and deformity.

osteoporosis A disease that causes bones to lose their mass and break easily.

osteotomy A surgical procedure involving the cutting of bone, usually performed in cases of severe joint malalignment.

pain A sensation or perception of hurting, ranging from discomfort to agony, that occurs in response to injury, disease or functional disorder. Pain is your body's alarm system, signaling that something is wrong. Acute pain, stemming from nerve endings stimulated by tissue damage, is temporary and improves with healing. Chronic pain may be mild to severe but persists due to prolonged tissue damage or pain impulses that keep the pain gate open.

palindromic rheumatism Self-limited attacks of joint inflammation that occur every few weeks or months, then subside after a few days. About one half of people who experience palindromic rheumatism go on to develop chronic rheumatoid arthritis.

pediatrician A physician with special training who specializes in the diagnosis, treatment and prevention of childhood and adolescent illness.

pediatric rheumatologist See rheumatologist.

peptic ulcer A benign (not cancerous) lesion in the stomach or duodenum that may cause pain, nausea, vomiting or bleeding. Such lesions can be caused by nonsteroidal anti-inflammatory drugs such as aspirin or ibuprofen.

pericarditis Inflammation of the lining surrounding the heart.

pharmacist A professional licensed to prepare and dispense drugs.

physiatrist A physician who continues training after medical school and specializes in the field of physical medicine and rehabilitation.

physical therapist A person who has professional training and is licensed in the practice of physical therapy.

physical therapy Methods and techniques of rehabilitation that help restore function and prevent disability following injury or disease. Methods may include applications of heat and cold, assistant devices, massage, and an individually tailored program of exercises.

physician A person who has successfully completed medical school and is licensed to practice medicine.

physician, family See physician, primary care.

physician, general practitioner See physician, primary care.

physician, primary care Physician to whom a family or individual goes initially when ill or for a periodic health check. The physician assumes medical coordination of care with other physicians for the patient with multiple health concerns.

physician's assistant A person trained, certified and licensed to assist physicians under the supervision by recording medical history and performing the physical examination, diagnosis and treatment of commonly encountered medical problems.

placebo effect The phenomenon in which a person receiving an inactive drug or therapy experiences a reduction in symptoms.

platelets Small cells that participate in the formation of blood clotting.

podagra Gout occurring in the big toe.

podiatrist A health professional who specializes in care of the foot. Formerly called a chiropodist.

polyarthritis Arthritis affecting many joints.

polymyositis Disease in which inflammation occurs primarily in the muscles, leading to muscle weakness and permanent muscle damage. Often associated with dermatomyositis, a condition marked by skin rashes.

proton pump inhibitors Drugs that block the secretion of acid into the stomach, used to protect the stomach against the gastrointestinal side effects associated with NSAIDs.

psoriatic arthritis A condition in which psoriasis (a common skin disease) occurs in conjunction with the inflammation of arthritis.

psychiatrist A physician who trains after medical school in the study, treatment and prevention of mental disorders. A psychiatrist may provide counseling and prescribe medicines and other therapies.

psychologist A trained professional, usually a PhD rather than an MD, who specializes in the mind and mental processes, especially in relation to human and animal behavior. A psychologist may measure mental abilities and provide counseling.

psychosomatic Pertaining to the link between the mind (psyche) and the body (soma).

pulmonary fibrosis Scarring of the lungs, leading to shortness of breath.

radiograph An X-ray.

range of motion (ROM) The distance and angles at which your joints can be moved, extended and rotated in various directions.

Raynaud's phenomenon Restriction of blood flow to the fingers, toes, or (rarely) to the nose or ears, in response to cold or emotional upset. This results in temporary blanching or paleness of the skin, tingling, numbness and pain.

reconditioning Restoring or improving muscle tone and strength with appropriate and balanced exercise, nutrition and rest. See also deconditioning.

rehabilitation counselor A person who guides physical and mental rehabilitation.

relaxation A state of release from mental or physical stress or tension.

remission The term used to describe a period when symptoms of a disease or condition improve or even disappear.

remodeling The regrowth of bone around an artificial joint.

resection Surgical procedure involving removing all or part of a bone.

resection arthroplasty A surgical procedure in which resection is done in conjunction with arthroplasty.

revision A surgical procedure to replace an artificial joint.

rheumatic disease A general term referring to conditions characterized by pain and stiffness of the joints or muscles. The American College of Rheumatology currently recognizes over 100 rheumatic diseases. The term is often used interchangeably with "arthritis" (meaning joint inflammation), but not all rheumatic diseases affect the joints or involve inflammation.

rheumatoid arthritis A chronic, inflammatory autoimmune disease in which the body's protective immune system turns on the body and attacks the joints, causing pain, swelling and deformity.

rheumatoid factor An abnormal antibody often found in blood of people with rheumatoid arthritis.

rheumatoid nodules Lumps of tissue that form under the skin, often over bony areas exposed to pressure, such as on the fingers or around the elbow.

rheumatologist A physician who pursues additional training after medical school and specializes in the diagnosis, treatment and prevention of arthritis and other rheumatic disorders.

rheumatologist, pediatric A rheumatologist who specializes in the diagnosis, treatment, and prevention of arthritis or other rheumatic diseases in children and adolescents.

salicylates A subcategory of NSAIDs, including aspirin.

scleritis Inflammation of the eyes.

scleroderma A connective tissue disease characterized by a tightening of the skin, and a discoloration of the hands when exposed to cold (known as Raynaud's phenomenon). Can affect internal organs as well.

scleromalacia perforans Permanent eye damage caused by severe inflammation

self-efficacy The concept of a person having emotional control in reaction to events in their life, such as a chronic illness.

self-help Any course, activity, or action that you do for yourself to improve your circumstances or ability to cope with a situation.

self-management The concept of a person having control of his or her disease and its management.

self-talk The voice in your head that you use to talk to yourself, aloud or in thought.

shared epitope Genetic marker that approximately two-thirds of people with rheumatoid arthritis have.

Sjögren's syndrome Syndrome affecting the salivary and lacrimal (tear-producing) glands, leading to dry eyes and dry mouth.

skeletal muscles The voluntary muscles that are involved primarily in moving parts of the body. "Voluntary" in this sense refers to muscles that move in response to our decisions to walk, bend, grasp, and so on, as opposed to muscles such as the heart, which do their work without our willful direction.

social worker A person who has professional training and is licensed to assist people in need by helping them capitalize on their own resources and connecting them with social services (for example, home nursing care or vocational rehabilitation).

soft-tissue rheumatism Pertaining to the many rheumatic conditions affecting the soft (as opposed to the hard or bony) tissues of the body. Fibromyalgia is one type of soft-tissue rheumatism. Others are bursitis, tendinitis and focal myofascial pain.

spontaneous remission A somewhat rare disappearance of symptoms of rheumatoid arthritis, usually occurring in the early stage of disease.

steroids A group name for lipids (fat substances) produced in the body and sharing a type of chemical structure. Among these are bile acids, cholesterol, and some hormones. Not the same as anabolic steroids, drugs synthesized from testosterone (the male sex hormone) and used by some athletes to promote strength and endurance.

strain Injury to a muscle, tendon or ligament by repetitive use, trauma or excessive stretching.

strengthening exercises Exercises that help maintain or increase muscle strength. See also isometric exercises and isotonic exercises.

stress The body's physical, mental and chemical reactions to frightening, exciting, dangerous or irritating circumstances.

stressor Factors that cause stress in your life.

symmetric arthritis Arthritis affecting the same joints on both sides of the body.

syndrome A collection of symptoms and/or physical findings that characterize a particular abnormal condition or illness.

synovectomy Surgical removal of the synovium, or the lining of the joint.

synovitis Inflammation of the lining of the joint.

synovium The lining of the joint.

synovial fluid The fluid found in the joint.

systemic disease A disease that may affect more than one system in the body.

target heart rate The number of heartbeats per minute to reach during exercise in order to gain maximum benefits. Because the normal heart rate changes as we age, target heart rates are grouped by age.

tendinitis Inflammation of a tendon.

tendon A cord of dense, fibrous tissue uniting a muscle to a bone.

TENS a treatment for pain involving a small device that directs mild electric pulses to nerves in the painful area.

teratogenic Causing the malformation of a fetus.

thrombocytopenia Decreased number of platelets.

tissue A collection of similar cells that act together to perform a specific function in the body. The primary tissues are epithelial (skin), connective (ligaments and tendons), bone, muscle and nerves.

titer A standard of strength per volume or units per volume.

trochanteric bursitis Irritation of the trochanteric bursa, which is located on the bony prominence of the femur or thigh. See also bursitis.

uric acid Substance formed when the body breaks down waste products called purines. Uric acid crystals deposited in the joints cause gout.

urinalysis Test done on the urine to detect levels of sugar, protein or abnormal cells.

vasculitis Inflammation of the blood vessels.

visual analogue scale A tool used to measure subjective feelings such as pain on a scale of 0 to 10 or 0 to 100.

visualization A method of imaginative thinking that allows you to picture achieving – and perhaps achieve – a goal.

warm-up Gentle movement to warm up the muscles before performing stretches and more strenuous exercise.

ADDITIONAL TERMS

ADDITIONAL TERMS

ADDITIONAL TERMS

NOTES

NOTES

NOTES

This section
contains
resources that
may be helpful
in managing
your health.

Resources

How You Can Use This Section:

This Resource section contains an overview of useful services and products offered by the Arthritis Foundation.

Find out how the Arthritis Foundation can help you learn more about your arthritis and how you can better manage it. Also find out how you can get involved with the Arthritis Foundation.

Use This Section to Record:

Additional Resources
Notes

Resources for Good Living

The Arthritis Foundation, the only national, voluntary health organization that works for the more than 46 million Americans with arthritis or chronic joint symptoms, offers many valuable resources through more than 150 offices nationwide. Your local office has information, products, classes and other services to help you take control of your arthritis or related condition. To find the chapter office nearest you, call 800-283-7800 or search the Arthritis Foundation Web site at www.arthritis.org.

Programs and Services

Physician referral
Most Arthritis Foundation chapters can provide a list of doctors in your area who specialize in the evaluation and treatment of arthritis and arthritis-related diseases.

Arthritis Programs
The Arthritis Foundation sponsors, develops and coordinates exercise programs for people with arthritis, featuring specially-trained instructors. They include:

1 **Arthritis Foundation Exercise Program** Relieve stiffness and lessen arthritis pain by doing low-impact exercises designed for people with arthritis and taught by trained instructors.

2 **Arthritis Foundation Aquatic Program** Join in the fun of a six- to 10-week exercise program in an heated pool led by trained instructors.

3 **Arthritis Foundation Self-Help Program** Learn how to take control of your own care in this six-week class for people with arthritis. This program was developed at Stanford University.

4 **Walk With Ease** This course allows participants to develop a walking plan that meets their individual needs, accompanied by the Arthritis Foundation book *Walk With Ease: Your Guide to Walking for Better Health, Improved Fitness and Less Pain*. A new audio walking guide is now available to use during your walking routines, with guidelines, upbeat music and inspiring motivation. In addition, a *Walk With Ease* group leader's manual is available to help you start and lead a walking group in your area.

5 **Tai Chi from the Arthritis Foundation** Developed by Dr. Paul Lam, the program consists of 12 movements — six basic and six advanced as well as a warm-up and cool-down.

Information and Products

Find the latest information about arthritis, including research, medications, government advocacy, programs and services through one of the many information resources offered by the Arthritis Foundation:

- **www.arthritis.org** Information about arthritis is available 24 hours a day on the Internet at the Arthritis Foundation's interactive, comprehensive Web site. Find news about arthritis, ways to get involved, and a variety of useful arthritis products, including books, brochures, videos and more.

- **Arthritis Answers** Call toll-free at 800-283-7800 for 24-hour, automated information about arthritis and Arthritis Foundation resources. Trained volunteers and staff are also available at your local Arthritis Foundation chapter to answer questions or refer you to physicians and other resources. Or e-mail questions to help@arthritis.org.

- **Books** The Arthritis Foundation publishes a variety of books on arthritis to help you learn to understand and manage your condition, live a healthier life, and cope with the emotional challenges that come with a chronic illness. Order books directly at www.arthritis.org or by calling 800-283-7800. All Arthritis Foundation books are available at your local bookstore.

- **Brochures** The Arthritis Foundation offers brochures containing concise, understandable information on the many arthritis-related diseases and conditions. Topics include surgery, the latest medications, guidance for working with your doctors and self-managing your illness. Single copies are available free of charge at www.arthritis.org or by calling 800-283-7800.

- *Arthritis Today* This award-winning bimonthly magazine provides the latest information on research, new treatments, trends and tips from experts and readers to help you manage arthritis. A one-year subscription to *Arthritis Today* is $12. A subscription is also included when you become a member of the Arthritis Foundation. Annual membership

is $20 and helps fund research to find cures for arthritis. Call 800-283-7800 for information.

- *Kids Get Arthritis Too* This newsletter focusing on juvenile rheumatic diseases, is published six times a year. Features speak to children and teens with the illness as well as to their parents. Stories examine the latest news in diagnosis, treatment and research of children's rheumatic diseases, as well as helpful ways kids can cope with their illnesses and the challenges they bring. This newsletter is free. To sign up, call 800-283-7800 or visit www.arthritis.org.

OTHER RESOURCES

OTHER RESOURCES

NOTES

NOTES

NOTES

NOTES

NOTES

NOTES

NOTES

NOTES

NOTES

NOTES

NOTES